I0429071

Diet in Relation to Age and Activity

Henry Thompson

Diet in Relation to Age and Activity

LM Publishers

I

Enough and more than enough, perhaps, has been uttered concerning the prejudicial effects on the body of habitually using alcoholic beverages. It is rare now to find any one, well acquainted with human physiology, and capable of observing and appreciating the ordinary wants and usages of life around him, who does not believe that, with few exceptions, men and women are healthier and stronger, physically, intellectually, and morally, without such drinks than with them. And confessedly there is little or nothing new to be said respecting a conclusion which has been so thoroughly investigated, discussed, and tested by experience, as this. It is useless, and indeed impolitic, in the well-intentioned effort to arouse public attention to the subject, to make exaggerated statements in relation thereto. But the important truth has still to be preached, repeated, and freshly illustrated, when possible, in every quarter of society, because a very natural bias to self-indulgence is always present to obscure's men views of those things which gratify it. While, in addition to this, an exceedingly clever commercial interest of enormous influence and proportions never ceases to vaunt its power to provide us with "the soundest," "purest," and most to be suspected of all with even "medically certified," forms of spirit, wine, and beer; apparently rendering alcoholic products conformable to the requirements of some physiological law supposed to demand their employment, and thus insinuating the semblance of a proof that they are generally valuable, or at least harmless, as an accompaniment of food at our daily meals.

It is not, however, with the evils of "drink" that I propose to deal here: they are thus alluded to because, in making a few observations on the kindred subject of food, I desire to commence with a remark on the comparison, so far as that is possible, between the deleterious effects on the body of erroneous views and practice in regard of drinking, and in regard of eating, respectively.

I have for some years past been compelled, by facts which are constantly coming before me, to accept the conclusion that more mischief in the form of actual disease, of impaired vigor, and of shortened life, accrues to civilized man, so far as I have observed in our own country and throughout Western and Central Europe, from erroneous habits in eating, than from the habitual use of alcoholic drink, considerable as I know the evil of that to be. I am not sure that a similar comparison might not be made between the respective influence of those agencies in regard of moral evil also; but I have no desire to indulge in speculative assertion, and suspect that an accurate conclusion on this subject may be beyond our reach at present.

It was the perception, during many years of opportunity to observe, of the extreme indifference manifested by the general public to any study of food, and want of acquaintance with its uses and value, together with a growing sense on my own part of the vast importance of diet to the healthy as well as to the sick, which led me in the year 1879 to write two articles in this review entitled "Food and Feeding." And since that date fresh experience has, I confess, still enhanced my estimate of the value of such knowledge, which indeed it is impossible to exaggerate, when regarding that one object of existence which I suppose all persons desire to attain, viz., an ample duration of time for enjoying the healthy exercise of bodily and mental function. Few would, I presume, consider length of life a boon apart from the possession of fairly good health; but this latter being granted, the desire for a prolonged term of existence appears to be almost universal.

I have come to the conclusion that a proportion amounting at least to more than one half of the disease which imbitters the middle and latter part of life among the middle and upper classes of the population is due to avoidable errors in diet. Further, while such disease renders so much of life, for many, disappointing, unhappy, and profitless, a term of painful endurance, for not a few it shortens life considerably. It would not be a difficult task—and its results if displayed here would be striking—to adduce in support of these views a numerical statement showing causes which prematurely terminate life among the classes referred to in this country, based upon the Registrar-General's reports, or by consulting the records of life-assurance experience. I shall not avail myself of these materials in this place, although it would be right to do so in the columns of a medical journal. My object here is to call the attention of the public to certain facts about diet which are insufficiently known, and therefore inadequately appreciated. And I shall assume that ample warrant for the observations made* here is within my reach, and can be made available if required.

At the outset of the few and brief remarks which the space at my disposal permits me to make, I shall intimate, speaking in general terms, that I have no sympathy with any dietary system which excludes the present generally recognized sources and varieties of food. It is possible, indeed, that we may yet add considerably to those we already possess, and with advantage; but there appears to be no reason for dispensing with anyone of them. When we consider how varied are the races of man, and how dissimilar are the climatic conditions which affect him, and how in each climate the occupations, the surrounding circumstances, and even the individual peculiarities of the inhabitants, largely differ, we shall be constrained to admit that any one of all the sources of food hitherto known may be made available, may in its turn become desirable, and even essential to life.

To an inhabitant of the Arctic Circle, for example, a vegetarian diet would be impracticable, because the elements of it cannot be produced in that region; and, were it possible to supply him with them, life could not be supported thereby. Animal food in large quantity is necessary to sustain existence in the low temperature to which he is exposed. But I desire to oppose any scheme for circumscribing the food resources of the world, and any form of a statute of limitations to our diet, not merely because it can be proved inapplicable, as in the case of the Esquimaux, under certain local and circumscribed conditions, but because I hold that the principle of limiting mankind to the use of any one class of foods among many is in itself an erroneous one. Thus, for example, while sympathizing to a large extent myself with the practice of what is called "vegetarianism" in diet, and knowing how valuable the exclusive or almost exclusive use of the products of the vegetable kingdom may be for a considerable number of the adult population of our own and of other countries in the temperate zones, and for most of that which inhabits the torrid zone, I object strongly to a dogmatic assertion that such limitation of their food is desirable for any class or body of persons whatever. Moreover, an exclusive or sectarian spirit always creeps in sooner or later, wherever an "ism" of any kind leads the way, which sooner or later brings in its train assertions barely supported by fact, the equivocal use of terms, evasion—in short, untruthfulness, unintended and unperceived by the well-meaning people who, having adopted the "ism," at last suffer quite unconsciously from obscurity of vision, and are in danger of becoming blind partisans.

Thus the term "vegetarian," as used to distinguish a peculiar diet, has no meaning whatever unless it implies that all the articles of food so comprised are to be products of the vegetable kingdom; admitting, of course, the very widest scope to that term. In that sense the vegetable kingdom may be held to embrace all the cereals, as wheat, barley, rye, and oats, maize, rice, and millet; all the leguminous plants—beans, peas, and lentils; all the roots and tubers containing chiefly starch, as the potato, yam, etc.; the plants yielding sago and arrowroot; the sources of sugar in the cane and beet, etc.; all the garden herbs and vegetables; the nuts, and all the fruits. Then there are the olive and other plants yielding the important element of oil in great abundance. An admirable assortment, to which a few minor articles belong, not necessary to be specified here. An excellent display of foods, which suffice to support life in certain favorable conditions, and which may be served in varied and appetizing forms. And to those who find their dietary within the limits of this list the name of vegetarian is rightly applicable. But such is by no means the practice of the self-styled vegetarians we usually meet with. It was only the other evening, in a crowded drawing-room, that a handsome, well-developed, and manifestly well-nourished girl—"a picture of health" and vigor—informed me with extreme satisfaction that she had been a "vegetarian" for several months, and how thoroughly that dietary system agreed with her. She added that she was recommending all her friends (how natural!) to be vegetarians also, continuing, "And do you not believe I am right?" On all grounds, one could only assure her that she had the appearance of admirably illustrating the theory of her daily life, whatever that might be, adding, "But now will you tell me what your diet consists of?" As happens in nineteen cases out of twenty, my young and blooming vegetarian replied that she took an egg and milk in quantity, besides butter, not only at breakfast, but again in the form of pudding, pastry, fritter, or cake, etc., to say nothing of cheese at each of the two subsequent meals of the day: animal food, it is unnecessary to say, of a choice, and some of it in a concentrated form. To call a person thus fed a vegetarian is a palpable error; to proclaim one's self so almost requires a stronger term to denote the departure from accuracy involved. Yet so attractive to some, possessing a moral sense not too punctilious, is the small distinction attained by becoming sectarian, and partisans of a quasi-novel and somewhat questioned doctrine, that an equivocal position is accepted in order to retain if possible the term "vegetarian" as the ensign of a party, the members of which consume abundantly strong animal food, abjuring it only in its grosser forms of flesh and fish. And hence it happens, as I have lately learned, that milk, butter, eggs, and cheese are now designated in the language of "vegetarianism" by the term "animal *products,*" an ingenious but evasive expedient to avoid the necessity for speaking of them as animal food!

Let us, for one moment only, regard milk, with which, on Nature's plan, we have all been fed for the first year, or thereabout, of our lives, and during which term we made a larger growth and a more important development than in any other year among the whole tale of the life which has passed, however long it may have been. How, in any sense, can that year of plenty and expansion, which we may have been happy and fortunate enough to owe—an inextinguishable debt—to maternal love and bounty, be said to be a year of "vegetarian diet"! Will any man henceforward dare thus to distinguish the source from which he drew his early life? Unhappily, indeed, for want of wisdom, the natural ration of some infants is occasionally supplemented at an early period by the addition of vegetable matter; but the practice is almost always undesirable, and is generally paid for by a sad and premature experience of indigestion to the helpless baby. Poor baby! who, unlike its progenitors in similar circumstances, while forced to pay the penalty, has not even had the satisfaction of enjoying a delightful but naughty dish beforehand.

The vegetarian restaurant at the Health Exhibition last summer supplied thousands of excellent and nutritious meals at a cheap rate, to the great advantage of its customers; but the practice of insisting with emphasis that a "vegetable diet" was supplied was wholly indefensible, since it contained eggs and milk, butter and cheese in great abundance.

It is not more than six months since I observed in a well-known weekly journal a list of some half-dozen receipts for dishes recommended on authority as specimens of vegetarian diet. All were savory combinations, and every one contained eggs, butter, milk, and cheese in considerable quantity, the vegetable elements being in comparatively small proportion!

It is incumbent on the supporters of this system of mixed diet to find a term which conveys the truth, that truth being that they abjure the use, as food, of all animal flesh. The words "vegetable" and "vegetarian" have not the remotest claim to express that fact, while they have an express meaning of their own in daily use – namely, the obvious one of designating products of the vegetable kingdom. It may not be easy at once to construct a simple term which differentiates clearly from the true vegetarian the person who also uses various foods belonging to the animal kigndom, and who abjures only the flesh of animals. But it is high time that we should be spared the obscure language, or rather the inaccurate statement, to which milk and egg consumers are committed, in assuming a title which has for centuries belonged to that not inconsiderable body of persons whose habits of life confer the right to use it. And I feel sure that my friends "the vegetarians," living on a mixed diet, will see the necessity of seeking a more appropriate designation to distinguish them; if not, we must endeavor to invent one for them.

But why should we limit by dogma or otherwise man's liberty to select his food and drink? I appreciate the reason for abstaining from alcoholic drinks derived from benevolent motive or religious principle, and entertain for it the highest respect, although I cannot myself claim the merit of self-denial or the credit of setting an example—abstaining, like many others, solely because experience has taught that to act otherwise is manifestly to do myself an injury.

This brings me to the point which I desire to establish, namely, that the great practical rule of life in regard of human diet will not be found in enforcing limitation of the sources of food which Nature has abundantly provided. On the contrary, that rule is fulfilled in the perfect development of the art of adapting food of any and every kind to the needs of the body according to the very varied circumstances of the individual, at different ages, with different forms of activity, with different inherent personal peculiarities, and with different environments. This may read at first sight, perhaps, like a truism; but how important is the doctrine, and how completely it is ignored in the experience of life by most people, it will be my object here to show.

I have already alluded to the fact that the young and rapidly growing infant, whose structures have to be formed on the soft and slender lines laid down before birth, whose organs have to be solidified and expanded at one and the same time, in which tissues of all kinds are formed with immense rapidity and activity, requires animal food ready prepared in the most soluble form for digestion and assimilation. Such a food is milk; and, if the human supply is insufficient, we obtain in its place that of the cow, chiefly; and during the first year of life milk constitutes the best form of food. After that time other kinds of nourishment, mostly well-cooked wheaten flour in various shapes, begin to be added to the milk which long continues to be a staple source of nourishment to the young animal. Eggs, a still more concentrated form of similar food, follow, and ultimately the dietary is enlarged by additions of various kinds, as the growing process continues through youth to puberty, when liberty arrives more or less speedily to do in all such matters "as others do." On reaching manhood, the individual in ninety-nine cases out of a hundred acquires the prevailing habit of his associates, and he feeds after that uniform prescription of diet which prevails, with little disposition to question its suitability to himself. A young fellow in the fullness of health, and habituated to daily active life in the open air, may, under the stimulus of appetite and enjoyment in gratifying it, often largely exceed both in quantity and variety of food what is necessary to supply all the demands of his system, without paying a very exorbitant price for the indulgence. If the stomach is sensitive or not very powerful, it sometimes rejects an extravagant ration of food, either at once or soon after the surfeit has been committed; but, if the digestive force is considerable, the meals, habitually superabundant as they may be, are gradually absorbed, and the surplus fund of nutrient material unused is stored up in some form.

When a certain amount has been thus disposed of, the capacity for storage varying greatly in different persons, an undesirable balance remains against the feeder, and in young people is mostly rectified by a "bilious attack," through the agency of which a few hours of vomiting and misery square the account. Then the same process of overfeeding recommences with renewed appetite and sensations of invigorated digestion, until in two or three, or five or six weeks, according to the ratio existing between the amount of food ingested and the habit of expending or eliminating it from the body, the recurring attack appears and again clears the system, and so on during several years of life. If the individual takes abundant exercise and expends much energy in the business of life, a large quantity of food can be properly disposed of. Such a person enjoys the pleasure of satisfying a healthy appetite, and doing so with ordinary prudence not only takes no harm, but consolidates the frame and enables it to resist those manifold unseen sources of evil which are prone to affect injuriously the feeble. On the other hand, if he is inactive, takes little exercise, spends most of his time in close air and in a warm temperature, shaping his diet nevertheless on the liberal scheme just described, the balance of unexpended nutriment soon tells more or less heavily against him, and must be thrown off in some form or another.

After the first half or so of life has passed away, instead of periodical sickness, the unemployed material may be relegated in the form of fat to be stored on the external surface of the body, or be packed among the internal organs, and thus he or she may become corpulent and heavy, if a facility for converting appropriate material into fat is consistent with the constitution of the individual; for some constitutions appear to be without the power of storing fat, however rich the diet or inactive their habits may be. When, therefore, this process cannot take place, and in many instances also when it is in action, the oversupply of nutritious elements ingested must go somewhere, more or less directly, to produce disease in some other form, probably at first interfering with the action of the liver, and next appearing as gout or rheumatism, or to cause fluxes and obstructions of various kinds. Thus recurring attacks of gout perform the same duty, or nearly so, at this period of life, that the bilious attacks accomplished in youth, only the former process is far more damaging to the constitution and materially injures it. In relation to liver derangement and inordinate fat production, we may see the process rapidly performed before our eyes, if we so desire, in the cellars of Strasburg. For the unfortunate goose who is made by force to swallow more nutritive matter than is good for him in the shape of food which, excellent in appropriate conditions, is noxious to the last degree when not expended by the consumer—I mean good milk and barley-meal—falls a victim in less than a month of this gluttonous living to that form of fatty liver which under the name of *foie gras* offers an irresistible charm to the gourmet at most well-furnished tables.

The animal being thus fed is kept in a close, warm temperature and without exercise, a mode of feeding and a kind of life which one need not after all go to Strasburg to observe, since it is not difficult to find an approach to it, and to watch the principle carried out, although only to a less considerable extent, anywhere and everywhere around us. Numerous individuals of both sexes, who have no claim by the possession of ornithological characteristics to consanguinity with the animal just named, may be said neverless to manifest signs of relation in some sort thereto—not creditable perhaps—to the goose, the Strasburg dietary being an enforced one—by their habit of absorbing superfluous quantities of nutriment while living a life of inactivity, and of course sooner or later become invalid in body, unhappy in temper, and decrepit in regard of mental power.

For let us observe that there are two forces concerned in this matter of bountiful feeding which must be considered a little further. I have said that a hearty, active young fellow may eat, perhaps, almost twice as much as he requires to replace the expenditure of his life and repair the loss of the machine in its working without much inconvenience. He, being robust and young, has two functions capable of acting at the maximum degree of efficiency. He has a strong digestion, and can convert a large mass of food into fluid aliment suitable for absorption into the system: that is function the first. But, besides this, he has the power of bringing into play an active eliminating force, which rids him of all the superfluous materials otherwise destined, as we have seen, to become mischievous in some shape: and that is function the second. To him it is a matter of indifference for a time whether the quantity of material which his food supplies to the body is greater than his ordinary daily expenditure demands, because his energy and activity furnish unstinted opportunities of eliminating the surplus at all times. But the neglect to adjust a due relation between the "income" and the "output" can not go on forever without signs of mischief in some quarter. A tolerably even correspondence between the two must by some means be maintained to insure a healthy condition of the body. It is failure to understand, first, the importance of preserving a near approach to equality between the supply of nutriment to the body and the expenditure produced by the activity of the latter, and, secondly, ignorance of the method of attaining this object in practice, which give rise to various forms of disease calculated to imbitter and shorten life after the period of prime has passed.

Let it be understood that in the matters of feeding and bodily activity a surplus of unexpended sustenance—here referred to as "the balance"—is by its nature exactly opposite to that which prudent men desire to hold with their bankers in affairs of finance. In this respect we desire to augment the income, endeavoring to confine expenditure within such limits as to maintain a cash balance in our favor to meet exigencies not perhaps foreseen. But, in order to preserve our health when that period of blatant, rampant, irrepressible vigor which belongs to youth has passed away, it is time to see that our income of food and our expenditure through such activity as we have constitute a harmonious equality, or nearly so. It is the balance against us of nutritive material which becomes a source of evil. And it is a balance which it is so agreeable and so easy to form, and which often so insidiously augments, unless we are on our guard against the danger. The accumulated stores of aliment, the unspent food, so to speak, which saturate the system are happily often got rid of by those special exercises to which so large a portion of time and energy is devoted by some people. It is to this end that men at home use dumb-bells or heavy clubs, or abroad shoot, hunt, and row, or perform athletic and pedestrian feats, or sweat in Turkish baths, or undergo a drench at some foreign watering-place—all useful exercises in their way, but pursued to an extent unnecessary for any other purpose than to eliminate superfluous nutrient materials, which are occasioning derangements in the system, for which these modes of elimination are the most efficient cure, and are thus often ordered by the medical adviser. But as we increase in age – when we have spent, say, our first half-century – less energy and activity remain, and less expenditure can be made; less power to eliminate is possible at fifty than at thirty, still less at sixty and upward. Less nutriment, therefore, must be taken in proportion as age advances, or rather as activity diminishes, or the individual will suffer. If he continues to consume the same abundant breakfasts, substantial lunches, and heavy dinners, which at the summit of his power he could dispose of almost with impunity, he will in time certainly either accumulate fat or become acquainted with gout or rheumatism, or show signs of unhealthy deposit of some kind in some part of the body, processes which must inevitably empoison, undermine, or shorten his remaining term of life. He must reduce his "intake," because a smaller expenditure is an enforced condition of existence.

At seventy the man's power has further diminished, and the nutriment must correspond thereto if he desires still another term of comfortable life. And why should he not? Then at eighty, with less activity there must be still less "support." And on this principle he may yet long continue, provided he is not the victim of an inherited taint or vice of system too powerful to be dominated, or that no unhappy accident inflicts a lasting injury on the machine, or no unfortunate exposure to insanitary poison has shaken the frame by long, exhausting fever; and then with a fair constitution he may remain free from serious troubles, and active to a right good old age, reaching far beyond the conventional seventy years which were formerly supposed to represent the full limit of man's fruitful life and work on earth.

But how opposed is this system to the favorite popular theory! Have we not all been brought up in the belief that the perfection of conduct consists, truly enough, in temperate habits in youth and middle life, such duty, however, being mostly enforced by the pleasant belief that when age arrived we might indulge in that extra "support"—seductive term, often fruitful of mischief—which the feebleness of advancing years is supposed to deserve? The little sensual luxuries, hitherto forbidden, now suggested by the lips of loving woman, and tendered in the confidence of well-doing by affectionate hands, are henceforth to be gratefully accepted, enjoyed, and turned to profit in the evening of our declining years. The extra glass of cordial, the superlatively strong extract of food, are now to become delicate and appropriate aids to the enfeebled frame. Unhappily for this doctrine, it is, on the contrary, precisely at this period that concentrated aliments are not advantageous or wholesome, but are to be avoided as sources generally prolific of trouble. If the cordial glass and the rich food are to be enjoyed at any time, whether prudently or otherwise, like other pleasures they must be indulged when strength and activity are great, in other words, when eliminating power is at its maximum, assuredly not when the circulation is becoming slow and feeble, and the springs of life are on the ebb. For the flow of blood cannot be driven into any semblance of the youthful torrent by the temporary force of stimulants, nor is it to be overcharged by the constant addition of rich elements which can no longer be utilized. And thus it is impossible to deny that an unsuspected source of discomfort, which in time may become disease, sometimes threatens the head of the household — a source which I would gladly pass over if duty did not compel me to notice it, owing as it is to the sedulous and tender care taken by the devoted, anxious partner of his life, who in secret has long noted and grieved over her lord's declining health and force. She observes that he is now more fatigued than formerly after the labors of the day, is less vigorous for business, for exercise, or for sport, less energetic every way in design and execution. She naturally desires to see him stronger, to sustain the enfeebled power which age is necessarily undermining; and with her there is but one idea, and it is practically embodied in one method — viz., to increase his force by augmenting his nourishment! She remonstrates at every meal at what she painfully feels is the insufficient portion of food he consumes. He pleads in excuse, almost with the consciousness of guilt, that he has really eaten all that appetite permits, but he is besought with plaintive voice and affectionate entreaty "to try and take a little more," and, partly to stay the current of gentle complaint, partly to gratify his companion, and partly, as with a faint internal sigh he may confess to himself, "for peace and comfort's sake," he assents, and with some violence to his nature forces his palate to comply, thus adding a slight burden to the already satiated stomach. Or if, perchance, endowed with a less compliant nature, he is churlish enough to decline the proffered advice, and even to question the value of a cup of strong beef-tea, or egg whipped up with sherry, which unsought has pursued him to his study, or been sent to his office between eleven and twelve of the forenoon, and which he knows by experience must if swallowed inevitably impair an appetite for lunch, then not improbably he will fall a victim to his solicitous helpmeet's well-meaning designs in some other shape. There is the tasteless calf's-foot jelly, of which a portion may be surreptitiously introduced into a bowl of tea with small chance that its presence will be detected, especially if accompanied by a good modicum of cream; or the little cup of cocoa or of coffee masking an egg well beaten and smoothly blended to tempt the palate—types of certain small diplomatic exercises, delightful, first, because they are diplomatic and not direct in execution; and, secondly, because the supporting system has been triumphantly maintained, my lord's natural and instinctive objections thereto notwithstanding.

But the loving wife – for whom my sympathy is not more profound than is my sorrow for her almost incurable error in relation to this single department of her duty—is by no means the only source of fallacious counsel to the man whose strength is slowly declining with age. We might almost imagine him to be the object of a conspiracy, so numerous are the temptations which beset him on every side. The daily and weekly journals display column after column of advertisements, enumerating all manner of edibles and drinkables, and loudly trumpeting their virtues, the chief of which is always declared to be the abundance of some quality averred to be at once medicinal and nutritious. Is it bread that we are conjured to buy? Then it is warranted to contain some chemical element; let it be, for example, "the phosphates in large proportion"—a mysterious term which the advertising tradesman has for some time past employed to signify a precious element, the very elixir of life, which somehow or other he has led the public to associate with the nutriment of the brain and nervous system, and vaunts accordingly. He has evidently caught the notion from the advertising druggist, who loudly declares his special forms of half-food, half-physic, or his medicated preparations of beef and mutton, to contain the elements of nutrition in the highest form of concentration, among which have mostly figured the aforesaid "phosphates"—as if they were not among the most common and generally prevalent of the earthy constituents of all our food! Then, lest haply a stomach, unaccustomed to the new and highly concentrated materials, should, as is not improbable, find itself unequal to the task of digesting and absorbing them, a portion of gastric juice, borrowed for the occasion, mostly from the pig, is associated therewith to meet, if possible, that difficulty, and so to introduce the nourishment by hook or by crook into the system. I don't say the method described may not be useful in certain cases, and on the advice of the experienced physician, for a patient exhausted by disease, whose salvation may depend upon the happy combination referred to. But it is the popular belief in the impossibility of having too much of that or of any such good thing, provided only it consists of nutritious food, that the advertiser appeals to, and appeals successfully, and with such effect that the credulous public is being gulled to an enormous extent. Then even our drink must now be nutritious! Most persons might naturally be aware that the primary object of drink is to satisfy thirst, which means a craving for the supply of water to the tissues—the only fluid they demand and utilize when the sensation in question is felt. Water is a solvent of solids, and is more powerful to this end when employed free from admixture with any other solid material. It may be flavored, as in tea and otherwise, without impairing its solvent power, but when mixed with any concrete matter, as in chocolate, thick cocoa, or even with milk, its capacity for dissolving—the very quality for which it was demanded—is in great part lost. So plentiful is nutriment in solid food, that the very last place where we should seek that quality is the drink which accompanies the ordinary meal. Here at least we might hope to be free from an exhortation to nourish ourselves, when desirous only to allay thirst or moisten our solid morsels with a draught of fluid. Not so; there are even some persons who must wash down their ample slices of roast beef with draughts of new milk!—an unwisely devised combination even for those of active habit, but for men and women whose lives are little occupied by exercise it is one of the greatest dietary blunders which can be perpetrated.

One would think it was generally known that milk is a peculiarly nutritive fluid, adapted for the fast-growing and fattening young mammal—admirable for such, for our small children, also serviceable to those whose muscular exertion is great, and, when it agrees with the stomach, to those who cannot take meat. For us who have long ago achieved our full growth, and can thrive on solid fare, it is altogether superfluous and mostly mischievous as a drink.

II

Another agent in the combination to maintain for the man of advancing age his career of flesh-eater is the dentist. Nothing is more common at this period of life than to hear complaints of indigestion experienced, so it is affirmed, because mastication is imperfectly performed for want of teeth. The dentist deftly repairs the defective implements, and the important function of chewing the food can be henceforth performed with comfort. But, without any intention to justify a doctrine of final causes, I would point out the significant fact that the disappearance of the masticating powers is mostly coincident with the period of life when that species of food which most requires their action—viz., solid animal fiber— is little, if at all, required by the individual. It is during the latter third of his career that the softer and lighter foods, such as well-cooked cereals, some light mixed animal and vegetable soups, and also fish, for which teeth are barely necessary, are particularly valuable and appropriate. And the man with imperfect teeth who conforms to Nature's demand for a mild, non-stimulating dietary in advanced years will mostly be blessed with a better digestion and sounder health than the man who, thanks to his artificial machinery, can eat and does eat as much flesh in quantity and variety as he did in the days of his youth. Far be it from me to undervalue the truly artistic achievements of a clever and experienced dental surgeon, or the comfort which he affords. By all means let us have recourse to his aid when our natural teeth fail, for the purpose of vocal articulation, to say nothing of their relation to personal appearance: on such grounds the artificial substitutes rank among the necessaries of life in a civilized community. Only let it be understood that the chief end of teeth, so far as mastication is concerned, has in advancing age been to a great extent accomplished, and that they are now mainly useful for the purposes just named. But I can not help adding that there are some grounds for the belief that those who have throughout life from their earliest years consumed little or no flesh, but have lived on a diet chiefly or wholly vegetarian, will be found to have preserved their teeth longer than those who have always made flesh a prominent part of their daily food.

Then there is that occasional visit to the tailor, who, tape in hand, announces in commercial monotone to the listening clerk the various measurements of our girth, and congratulates us on the gradual increase thereof. He never in his life saw you looking so well, and "fancy, sir, you are another inch below your armpits"—a good deal below—"since last year!" insidiously intimating that in another year or so you will have nearly as fine a chest as Heenan! And you, poor deluded victim, are more than half willing to believe that your increasing size is an equivalent to increasing health and strength, especially as your wife emphatically takes that view, and regards your augmenting portliness with approval. Ten years have now passed away since you were forty, and by weight twelve stone and a half a fair proportion for your height and build. Now you turn the scale to one stone more, every ounce of which is fat; extra weight to be carried through all the labors of life. If you continue your present dietary and habits, and live five or seven years more, the burden of fat will be doubled; and that insinuating tailor will be still congratulating you. Meantime you are "running the race of life"—a figure of speech less appropriate to you at the present moment than it formerly was—handicapped by a weight which makes active movement difficult, upstair ascents troublesome, respiration thick and panting. Not one man in fifty lives to a good old age in this condition. The typical man of eighty or ninety years, still retaining a respectable amount of energy of body and mind, is lean and spare, and lives on slender rations. Neither your heart nor your lungs can act easily and healthily, being oppressed by the gradually gathering fat around. And this because you continue to eat and drink as you did, or even more luxuriously than you did, when youth and activity disposed of that moiety of food which was consumed over and above what the body required for sustenance. Such is the import of that balance of unexpended aliment which your tailor and your foolish friends admire, and the gradual disappearance of which, should you recover your senses and diminish it, they will still deplore, half frightening you back to your old habits again by saying, "You are growing thin: *what can be the matter with you?*" Insane and mischievous delusion!

It is interesting to observe that the principle I have thus endeavored to illustrate and support, little as it is in accordance with the precept and practice of modern authority, was clearly enunciated so long ago as the sixteenth century. The writings of Luigi Cornaro, who was born of noble family in Venice soon after the middle of the fifteenth century, and was contemporary for seventy years with Titian, wrote his first essay on the subject of regimen and diet for the aged when eighty-three years of age, producing three others during the subsequent twelve years. His object was to show that, with increasing age and diminished powers, a corresponding decrease in the quantity of food must be taken in order to preserve health. He died at Padua "without any agony, sitting in an elbow-chair, being above one hundred years old."

Thus he writes:

There are old lovers of feeding who say that it is necessary they should eat and drink a great deal to keep up their natural heat, which is constantly diminishing as they advance in years; and that it is, therefore, their duty to eat heartily, and of such things as please their palate, be they hot, cold, or temperate; and that, were they to lead a sober life, it would be a short one. To this I answer that our kind mother, Nature, in order that old men may live still to a greater age, has contrived matters so that they should be able to subsist on little, as I do, for large quantities of food cannot be digested by old and feeble stomachs.... By always eating little the stomach, not being much burdened, need not wait long to have an appetite. It is for this reason that dry bread relishes so well with me; and I know it from experience, and can with truth affirm, I find such sweetness in it that I should be afraid of sinning against temperance, were it not for my being convinced of the absolute necessity of eating of it, and that we cannot make, use of a more natural food. And thou, kind parent Nature, who actest so lovingly by thy aged offspring, in order to prolong his days, hast contrived mattters so in his favor, that he can live upon very little; and, in order to add to the favor, and do him still greater service, hast made him sensible, that as in his youth he used to eat twice a day, when he arrives at old age he ought to divide that food, of which he was accustomed before to make but two meals, into four; because, thus divided, it will be more easily digested; and, as in his youth he made but two collations in the day, he should, in his old age, make four, provided, however, he lessens the quantity as his years increase.

And this is what I do, agreeably to my own experience; and, therefore, my spirits, not oppressed by much food, but barely kept up, are always brisk, especially after eating, so that I am obliged then to sing a song, and afterward to write.

Nor do I ever find myself the worse for writing immediately after meals, nor is my understanding ever clearer, nor am I apt to be drowsy, the food I take being in too small a quantity to send up any fumes to the brain. Oh, how advantageous it is to an old man to eat but little! Accordingly I, who know it, eat but just enough to keep body and soul together.

Cornaro ate of all kinds of food, animal as well as vegetable, but in very small quantity, and he drank moderately of the light wine of his country, diminishing his slender rations as age increased. I am quite aware that I am reciting a story which must be familiar to some of the readers of this review. But it is by no means widely known, and is too apt an example of the value of the law under consideration not to be referred to here.

It must now be clearly understood, as a general rule for men at all ages, that the amount of food ingested ought to accord within certain narrow limits with the amount of force employed for the purposes of daily life. But there is a certain qualification, apparent but not real, of the principle thus enunciated which must be referred to here, in order to prevent misunderstanding or misinterpretation of my meaning in relation to one particular. It is right and fitting that a certain amount of storage material, or balance, should exist as a reserve in the constitution of every healthy man. Every healthy individual, indeed, necessarily possesses a stored amount of force, which will stand him in good stead when a demand arises for prolonged unusual exertion, or when any period of enforced starvation occurs, as during a lingering fever or other exhausting disease. The existence of this natural and healthy amount of reserved force is of course presupposed throughout all my remarks, and its extreme value is taken for granted. That undue amount of stored nutriment, that balance which has been referred to as prejudicial to the individual, is a quantity over and above the natural reserve produced by high health; for, when augmented beyond that point, the material takes the form of diseased deposit, and ceases to be an available source of nutriment. Even the natural amount of store or reserve is prone to exceed the necessary limit in those who are healthy or nearly so. Hence it is that in all systems of training for athletic exploits—

which is simply a process of acquiring the highest degree of health and strength attainable, in view of great or prolonged exertion—some loss of weight is almost invariably incurred in developing a perfect condition. In other words, almost any man who sets himself to acquire by every means in his power the best health possible for his system does in the process necessary thereto throw off redundant materials, the presence of which is not consistent with the high standard of function required. Thus what is sometimes called "overtraining" is a condition in which the storage is reduced too much, and some weakening is incurred thereby; while "undertraining" implies that the useless fatty and other matters have not been sufficiently got rid of, so that the athlete is encumbered by unnecessary weight, and is liable to needless embarrassments, telling against his chances in more ways than one. The exact and precise balance between the two conditions is the aim of the judicious trainer.

We are thus led to the next important consideration, namely, that although broad rules or principles of diet may be enunciated as applicable to different classes of people in general, no accurate adaptation to the individual is possible without a knowledge of his daily habits and life, as well as to some extent of his personal peculiarities. No man, for example, can tell another what he can or ought to eat, without knowing what are the habits of life and work—mental and bodily—of the person to be advised. Notwithstanding which, no kind of counsel is more frequently tendered in common conversation by one stranger with another, than that which concerns the choice of food and drink. The adviser feels himself warranted, by the experience that some particular combination of nourishment suits his own stomach, to infer without hesitation that this dish will be therefore acceptable to the stomachs of all his neighbors. Surely the intelligence of such a man is as slender as his audacity and presumption are large. It would not he more preposterous if, having with infinite pains obtained a last representing precisely the size and the peculiarities in form of his own foot, he forthwith solemnly adjured all other persons to adopt boots made upon that model, and on none other! Only it may be assumed that there is probably more difference between stomachs and their needs among different individuals than among the inferior extremities referred to for the purpose of illustration. Thus, in regard of expenditure of food, how great is the difference between that of a man who spends ten or twelve hours of the day at the work of a navvy, as an agricultural laborer in harvest-time, or in draining or trenching land, as a sawyer, a railway porter, or a bricklayer's laborer, or let me add that of an ardent sportsman, as compared with the expenditure of a clerk who is seated at the desk, of individuals engaged in literary and artistic pursuits, demanding a life mostly sedentary and spent indoors, with no exercise but that which such persons voluntarily take as a homage to hygienic duty, and for a short period borrowed at some cost from engagements which claim most of their time and nearly all their energies! While the manual laborers rarely consume more food than they expend, and are, if not injured by drink, or by undue exposure to the weather, mostly hale and hearty in consequence, the latter are often martyrs to continued minor ailments, which gradually increase, and make work difficult, and life dreary. Few people will believe how easy it is in most instances to meet the difficulty by adopting appropriate food, and that such brain-workers can really enjoy a fair degree of health and comfort by living on light food, which does not require much force to digest, and much muscular activity to assimilate—a diet, moreover, which is important to some of these from another point of view—the financial one—inasmuch as it is at least less costly by one half than the conventional meals which habit or custom prescribes alike to large classes of men in varied conditions of life. But there is another and more important economic gain yet to be named, as realizable through the use of a light and simple dietary. It is manifested by the fact that a greater expenditure of nerve-power is demanded for the digestion of heavy meat meals than for the lighter repasts which are suitable to the sedentary; from which fact it results of course that this precious power is reserved for more useful and more delightful pursuits than that of mere digestion, especially when this is not too well performed.

But those who have little time for exercise, and are compelled to live chiefly within-doors, must endeavor to secure, or should have secured for them as far as possible by employers, by way of compensation, a regular supply of fresh air without draughts, an atmosphere as free from dust and other impurities as can be obtained, with a good supply of light, and some artificial warmth when needed. These necessities granted, cereal foods, such as well-made bread in variety, and vegetable produce, including fruits, should form a great part of the diet consumed, with a fair addition of eggs and milk if no meat is taken, and little of other animal food than fish. On such a dietary, and without alcoholic stimulants, thousands of such workers as I have briefly indicated may enjoy with very little exercise far better health and more strength than at present they experience on meat and heavy puddings, beer, baker's bread, and cheese. Of course there are workers who belong to neither of the two extreme classes indicated, and whose habits cannot be described as sedentary, but who occupy a middle place between the two. For such, some corresponding modification of the dietary is naturally appropriate. But it is a vulgar error to regard meat in any form as necessary to life; if for any it is necessary, it is for the hard-working out-door laborers above referred to, and for these a certain proportion is no doubt desirable. Animal flesh is useful also as a concentrated form of nutriment, valuable for its portability; and, for the small space it occupies in the stomach, unrivaled in certain circumstances. Like every other description of food, it is highly useful in its place, but is by no means necessary for a large proportion of the population. To many it has become partially desirable only by the force of habit, and because their digestive organs have thus been trained to deal with it, and at first resent a change. But, this being gradually made, adaptation takes place, and the individual who has consumed two or three meat meals daily with some little discomfort, chiefly from being often indisposed to make active exertions, becomes, after sufficient time has elapsed, stronger, lighter, and happier, as well as better tempered, and manifestly healthier, on the more delicate dietary sketched. People in general have very inadequate ideas of the great power of habit alone in forming what they believe to be innate personal peculiarities, or in creating conditions which are apparently part of a constitutional necessity, laws of their nature and essential to their existence. Many of these peculiarities are solely due to habit, that is, to long continuance in a routine of action, adopted it may be without motive or design; and people are apt to forget that, if a routine of a precisely opposite character had been adopted, precisely opposite conditions would have been established, and opposite peculiarities would have become dominant, as their contraries are now. Alterations in the dietary, especially of elderly persons, should be made gradually and with caution. This condition fulfilled, a considerable change may be effected with satisfactory results, when circumstances render it necessary. To revert once more to the question of flesh-eating, it should be remarked that it appears to be by no means a natural taste with the young. Few children like that part of the meal which consists of meat, but prefer the pudding, the fruit, the vegetables, if well dressed, which unhappily is not often the case.

Many children manifest great repugnance to meat at first, and are coaxed and even scolded by anxious mothers until the habit of eating it is acquired. Adopting the insular creed, which regards beef and mutton as necessary to health and strength, the mother often suffers from groundless forebodings about the future of a child who rejects flesh, and manifests what is regarded as an unfortunate partiality for bread and butter and pudding. Nevertheless, I am satisfied, if the children followed their own instinct in that matter, the result would be a gain in more ways than one. Certainly, if meat did not appear in the nursery until the children sent for it, it would be rarely seen there, and the young ones would as a rule thrive better on milk and eggs, with the varied produce of the vegetable kingdom.

A brief allusion must be made to the well-known and obvious fact that the surrounding temperature influences the demand for food, which therefore should be determined as regards quantity or kind according to the climate inhabited, or the season of the year as it affects each climate. In hot weather, the dietary should be lighter, in the understood sense of the term, than in cold weather. The sultry period of our summer, although comparatively slight and of short duration, is nevertheless felt by some persons to be extremely oppressive; but this is mainly due to the practice of eating much animal food or fatty matters, conjoined as it often is with the habit of drinking freely of fluids containing a small quantity of alcohol. Living on cereals, vegetables, and fruits, with some proportion of fish, and abstaining from alcoholic drinks, the same person would probably enjoy the high temperature, and be free from the thirst which is the natural result of consuming needlessly substantial and heating food.

There is a very common term, familiar by daily use, conveying unmistakably to everyone painful impressions regarding those who manifest the discomforts indicated by it - I mean the term indigestion. The first sign of what is so called may appear even in childhood; not being the consequence of any stomach disorder, but solely of some error in diet, mostly the result of eating too freely of rich compounds in which sugar and fatty matters are largely present. These elements would not be objectionable if they formed part of a regular meal, instead of being consumed as they mostly are between meals, already abounding in every necessary constituent.

Sugar and fat are elements of value in children's food, and naturally form a considerable portion of it, entering largely into the composition of milk, which Nature supplies for the young and growing animal. The indigestion of the child mostly terminates rapidly by ejection of the offending matter. But the indigestion of the adult is less acutely felt and is less readily disposed of. Uneasiness and incapacity for action, persisting for some time after an ordinary meal, indicate that the stomach is acting imperfectly on the materials which have been put into it. These signs manifest themselves frequently, and, if Nature's hints that the food is inappropriate are not taken, they become more serious. Temporary relief is easily obtained by medicine; but if the unfortunate individual continues to blame his stomach, and not the dietary he selects, the chances are that his troubles will continue, or appear in some other form. At length, if unenlightened on the subject, he becomes "a martyr to indigestion," and resigns himself to the unhappy fate, as he terms it, of "the confirmed dyspeptic."

Such a victim may perhaps be surprised to learn that nine out of ten persons so affected are probably not the subjects of any complaint whatever, and that the stomach at any rate is by no means necessarily faulty in its action—in short, that what is popularly termed "indigestion" is rarely a disease in any sense of the word, but merely the natural result of errors in diet. For most men it is the penalty of conformity to the eating habits of the majority; and a want of disposition or of enterprise to undertake a trial of simpler foods than those around them consume probably determines the continuance of their unhappy troubles. In many instances it must be confessed that the complaint, if so it must be called, results from error, not in the quality of the food taken, but in the quantity. Eating is an agreeable process for most people, and under the influence of very small temptation, or through undue variety furnishing a source of provocation to the palate, a considerable proportion of nutritious material above what is required by the system is apt to be swallowed. Then it is also to be remembered that stomachs which vary greatly in their capacity and power to digest may all nevertheless be equally healthy and competent to exercise every necessary function. In like manner we know that human brains which are equally sound and healthy often differ vastly in power and in activity. Thus a stomach, which would be slandered by a charge of incompetence to perform easily all that it is in duty bound to accomplish, may be completely incapable of digesting a small excess beyond that natural limit. Hence, with such an organ an indigestion is inevitable when this limit is only slightly exceeded. And so when temptations are considerable, and frequently complied with, the disturbance may be, as it is with some, very serious in degree. How very powerful a human stomach may sometimes be, and how large a task in the way of digestion it may sometimes perform without complaint, is known to those who have had the opportunity of observing what certain persons with exceptional power are accustomed to take as food, and do take for a long time apparently with impunity. But these are stomachs endowed with extraordinary energy, and woe be to the individual with a digestive apparatus of moderate power who attempts to emulate the performance of a neighbor at table who perchance may be furnished with such an effective digestive apparatus!

But, after all, let not the weaker man grieve overmuch at the uneven lot which the gods seem to have provided for mortals here below in regard of this function of digestion. There is a compensation for him which he has not considered, or perhaps even heard of, although he is so moderately endowed with peptic force. A delicate stomach which can just do needful work for the system and no more, by necessity performs the function of a careful door porter at the entrance of the system, and like a jealous guardian inspects with discernment all who aspire to enter the interior, rejecting the unfit and the unbidden, and all the common herd.

On the other hand, a stomach with superfluous power, of whom its master boastfully declaims that it can "digest tenpenny nails," and that he is unaccustomed to consult its likes and its dislikes if it have any, is like a careless hall porter who admits all comers, every pretender, and among the motley visitors many whose presence is damaging to the interior. These powerful feeders after a time suffer from the unexpended surplus, and pay for their hardy temerity in becoming amenable to penalty, often suddenly declared by the onset of some serious attack, demanding complete change in regimen, a condition more or less grave. On the other hand, the owner of the delicate stomach, a man perhaps with a habit of frequently complaining of slight troubles, and always careful, will probably in the race of life, as regards the preceding pilgrim, take the place of the tortoise as against the hare. It is an old proverb that "the creaking wheel lasts longest," and one that is certainly true as regards a not powerful but nevertheless healthy stomach which is carefully treated by its owner; to whom this fact may be acceptable as a small consolation for the possession of a delicate organ.

For it is a kind of stomach which not seldom accompanies a fine organization. The difference is central, not local—a difference in the nervous system chiefly; the impressionable mental structure, the instrument of strong emotions, must necessarily be allied with a stomach to which the supply of nerve-power for digestion is sometimes temporarily deficient and always perhaps capricious. There are more sources than one of compensation to the owner of an active, impressionable brain, with a susceptible stomach possessing only moderate digestive capabilities—sources altogether beyond the imagination of many a coarse feeder and capable digester.

But it is not correct, and it is on all grounds undesirable, to regard the less powerful man as a sufferer from indigestion, that is, as liable to any complaint to be so termed. True indigestion, as a manifestation of a diseased stomach, is comparatively quite rare, and I have not one word to say of it here, which would not be the fitting place if I had. Not one person in a hundred who complains of indigestion has any morbid affection of the organs engaged in assimilating his food. As commonly employed, the word "indigestion" denotes, not a disease, but an admonition. It means that the individual so complaining has not yet found his appropriate diet; that he takes food unsuited for him, or too much of it. The food may be "wholesome enough in itself," a popular phrase permitted to appear here, first, because it conveys a meaning perceived by everyone, although the idea is loosely expressed; but, secondly and chiefly, for the purpose of pointing out the fallacy which underlies it. There is no food "wholesome in itself," and there is no fact which people in general are more slow to comprehend. That food only is wholesome which is so to the individual, and no food can be wholesome to any given number of persons. Milk, for example, may agree admirably with me, and may as certainly invariably provoke an indigestion from my neighbor; and the same may be said of almost every article of our ordinary dietary. The wholesomeness of a food consists solely in its adaptability to the individual, and this relation is governed mainly by the influences of his age, activity, surroundings and temperament or personal peculiarities.

Indigestion, therefore, does not necessarily, or indeed often, require medicine for its removal. Drugs, and especially small portions of alcoholic spirit, are often used for the purpose of stimulating the stomach temporarily to perform a larger share of work than by nature it is qualified to undertake; a course which is disadvantageous for the individual if persisted in. The effect on the stomach is that of the spur on the horse: it accelerates the pace, but "it takes it out" of the animal, and, if the practice is long continued, shortens his natural term of efficiency.

It is an erroneous idea that a simple form of dietary, such as the vegetable kingdom in the largest sense of the term furnishes, in conjunction with a moderate proportion of the most easily digested forms of animal food, may not be appetizing and agreeable to the palate. On the contrary, I am prepared to maintain that it may be easily served in forms highly attractive, not only to the general but to a cultivated taste. A preference for the high flavors and stimulating scents peculiar to the flesh of vertebrate animals mostly subsides after a fair trial of milder foods when supplied in variety. And it is an experience almost universally avowed, that the desire for food is keener, that the satisfaction in gratifying appetite is greater and more enjoyable, on the part of the general light feeder than with the almost exclusively flesh-feeder. For this designation is applicable to almost all those who compose the middle-class population of this country. They consume little bread and few vegetables; all the savory dishes are of flesh, with decoctions of flesh alone for soup. The sweets are compounds of suet, lard, butter, eggs and milk, with very small quantities of flour, rice, arrowroot, etc., which comprise all the vegetable constituents besides some fruit and sugar. Three fourths at least of the nutrient matters consumed are from the animal kingdom. A reversal of the proportions named, that is, a fourth only from the latter source with three fourths of vegetable produce, would furnish greater variety for the table, tend to maintain a cleaner palate, increased zest for food, a lighter and more active brain, and a better state of health for most people not engaged on the most laborious employments of active life; while even for the last named, with due choice of material, ample sustenance in the proportions named may be supplied. For some inactive, sedentary, and aged persons the small proportion of animal food indicated might be advantageously diminished. I am frequently told by individuals of sixty years and upward that they have no recollection of any previous period since reaching mature age at which they have possessed a keener relish for food than that which they enjoy at least once or twice a day since they have adopted the dietary thus described. Such appetite at all events as has rarely offered itself during years preceding, when the choice of food was conventionally limited to the unvarying progression and array of mutton and beef, in joint, chop, and steak, arriving after a strong meat soup, with a possible interlude of fish, and followed by puddings of which the ingredients are chiefly derived from animal sources. The penetrating odors of meat cookery which announce their presence by escape from the kitchen, and will pervade the air of other rooms in any private house but a large one, and which are encountered in clubs, restaurants, and hotels without stint, alone suffice to blunt the inclination for food of one who, returning from daily occupation, fatigued and fastidious, desires food easy of digestion, attractive in appearance, and unassociated with any element of a repulsive character. The light feeder knows nothing of the annoyances described, finds on his table that which is delightful to a palate sensitive to mild impressions, and indisposed to gross and over-powerful ones. After the meal is over, his wit is fresher, his temper more cheerful, and he takes his easychair to enjoy fireside talk, and not to sink into a heavy slumber, which on awakening is but exchanged for a sense of discontent or stupidity.

The doctrine thus briefly and inadequately expounded in this paper may probably encounter some opposition and adverse criticism. I am quite content that this should be so. Every proposal which disturbs the current habits of the time, especially when based on long-prevalent custom, infallibly encounters that fate. But of the general truth, and hence of the ultimate reception of the principles I have endeavored to illustrate, there cannot be the faintest doubt. And I know that this result, whenever it may be accomplished, will largely diminish the painful affections which unhappily so often appear during the latter moiety of adult life. And having during the last few years widely inculcated such general dietetic principles and practice, with abundant grounds for my growing conviction of their value, it appears to be a duty to call attention to them somewhat more emphatically than in preceding contributions already referred to. In so doing I have expressly limited myself to statements relating to those simple elementary facts concerning our every-day life which ought to be within the knowledge of every man, and therefore such as may most fitly be set forth in a publication outside of that field of special and technical record which is devoted to professional observation and experience.